VALERIE HEPBURN

Gluten Etiquette

Navigating Social Spaces with Gluten-Sensitive Friends

First edition

This book was professionally typeset on Reedsy.
Find out more at reedsy.com

Contents

Introduction

Purpose of This Guide

This guide is designed to help anyone new to dealing with a gluten allergy, whether it's yourself or a loved one. There are many best practices that are not difficult to follow, you just need to know the basics and then commit to implementing them for the safety of yourself or your friend.

Discovering that a friend has a gluten allergy can be a transformative moment in your relationship. As you embark on this journey together, it's crucial to understand the challenges and nuances of living with gluten sensitivity. In this guide, we will explore various aspects of supporting your friend with a gluten allergy, from understanding the condition to practical tips for creating a gluten-friendly environment.

Supporting a friend with a gluten allergy requires a blend of understanding, empathy, and practical assistance. By educating yourself, creating a gluten-friendly environment, facilitating positive social experiences, and being there during challenging times, you can contribute significantly to your friend's well-being. Remember that this journey is a partnership, and your commitment to understanding and accommodating their needs will strengthen your friendship while enhancing their quality of life. And you will have fun along the way learning together.

Chapter 1 - Basic Knowledge

Understanding Gluten Allergy

Before diving into the ways you can support your friend, it's essential to grasp the fundamentals of gluten allergy. Gluten is a protein found in wheat, barley, rye, and their derivatives. Individuals with gluten sensitivity or celiac disease experience adverse reactions when they consume gluten, leading to a range of symptoms from digestive issues, and skin problems to neurological concerns. By familiarizing yourself with the basics, you can better empathize with and support your friend's challenges.

Educate Yourself

One of the most powerful ways to support a friend with a gluten allergy is to educate yourself about the condition. Understanding the impact of gluten on your friend's health will enable you to make informed decisions and provide better support.

Empathize and Listen

Living with a gluten allergy can be emotionally and physically taxing. Be a compassionate listener when your friend wants to share their experiences, frustrations, or fears related to their dietary restrictions. Sometimes, all they need is someone who understands and empathizes with their journey. Avoid offering unsolicited advice unless your friend explicitly asks for it, as this can be overwhelming.

Celiac Disease vs Gluten Sensitivity

Celiac Disease:

Celiac Disease is an autoimmune disorder triggered by the ingestion of gluten – a protein found in wheat, barley, and rye. In individuals with Celiac Disease, the immune system mistakenly identifies gluten as a threat and launches an attack on the small intestine, damaging the delicate villi that line its walls. These finger-like projections are crucial for nutrient absorption, and their impairment can lead to malabsorption issues and various symptoms. People with celiac disease have a 2x greater risk of developing coronary artery disease, and a 4x greater risk of developing small bowel cancers.

Untreated celiac disease can lead to the development of other autoimmune disorders like type 1 diabetes and multiple sclerosis (MS), and many other conditions, including dermatitis herpetiformis (an itchy skin rash), anemia, osteoporosis, intestinal cancers, infertility and miscarriage, neurological conditions like epilepsy and migraines and heart disease.

Gluten Sensitivity:

Gluten Sensitivity, also known as Non-Celiac Gluten Sensitivity (NCGS), is a more loosely defined condition. Unlike Celiac Disease, Gluten Sensitivity does not involve an autoimmune response or result in the characteristic intestinal damage seen in Celiac patients. Instead, individuals with Gluten Sensitivity experience a range of symptoms after consuming gluten, without the autoimmune component. Common Symptoms will be covered next.

Why Does All This Matter?

It matters because the consequences of ingesting gluten for a person with Celiac Disease or Gluten Sensitivity can be severe. The symptoms can affect the quality of life and longevity of a person, especially if not contained to a few accidental contacts throughout their life. The severity of any given symptom will vary from person to person. Sometimes it's a minor temporary inconvenience, sometimes it will change the course of someone's life, especially the neurological and gastrointestinal expressions.

Chapter 2 - Common Symptoms

Gastrointestinal Symptoms

Abdominal Discomfort: Individuals with gluten allergies often experience bloating, gas, and abdominal pain after consuming gluten-containing foods. This discomfort may vary in intensity but is a recurring issue for those with gluten sensitivity.

Diarrhea or Constipation: Gluten sensitivity can disrupt normal bowel function, leading to episodes of diarrhea or constipation. These symptoms may be sporadic but are often linked to gluten consumption.

Nausea and Vomiting: Some individuals may feel nauseous or experience vomiting after ingesting gluten, further emphasizing the intricate relationship between gluten and the digestive system.

Neurological Symptoms

Cognitive Impairment: Cognitive impairment refers to a condition in which a person's cognitive abilities are diminished or compromised. Cognitive abilities include various mental processes such as memory, attention, language, problem-solving, and executive function. Cognitive impairment can range from mild to severe and can affect different aspects of a person's daily life.

Headaches or Migraines: Gluten sensitivity can trigger chronic headaches or migraines in some individuals. The connection between gluten and headaches is not fully understood, but many report relief from their symptoms upon adopting a gluten-free diet.

Brain Fog: Cognitive symptoms such as difficulty concentrating, memory issues, and a feeling of mental fogginess are frequently reported by those with gluten allergies. This phenomenon is commonly referred to as "brain fog."

Fatigue: Fatigue is a state of extreme tiredness and lack of energy, both physically and mentally. It goes beyond normal tiredness and often results in a persistent feeling of exhaustion that can interfere with daily activities and functioning. Physical fatigue may manifest as weakness, aches, and a reduced capacity for physical tasks.

Mood Changes: Gluten sensitivity may contribute to mood swings, anxiety, rage, or depression. Research suggests a potential link between gluten and the central nervous system, impacting mood regulation.

Skin Issues

Dermatitis Herpetiformis: In some cases, gluten sensitivity can manifest as dermatitis herpetiformis, a chronic skin condition characterized by itchy, blistering rashes. This condition is linked to celiac disease but can also occur in the absence of intestinal symptoms.

Eczema and Psoriasis: Gluten sensitivity has been associated with exacerbating existing skin conditions such as eczema and psoriasis. Managing gluten intake may contribute to alleviating these skin issues for some individuals.

Chapter 3 - What is Gluten?

Gluten is a mixture of proteins found in wheat and related grains, such as barley, rye, and oats. It is primarily composed of two proteins: glutenin and gliadin. Gluten gives dough its elasticity and helps it rise by trapping gases produced during fermentation, contributing to the structure and texture of baked goods.

While gluten is a key component in many staple foods like bread, pasta, and pastries, some people need to avoid it due to gluten-related disorders. Celiac disease is an autoimmune disorder in which the ingestion of gluten leads to damage in the small intestine. Non-celiac gluten sensitivity is another condition where individuals experience gastrointestinal and/or extra-intestinal symptoms after consuming gluten but without the autoimmune response seen in celiac disease.

For those without gluten-related issues, gluten is generally safe and provides an essential dietary component. However, it's important to be aware of gluten content for individuals with gluten-related disorders or those following a gluten-free diet for other reasons.

Wheat and Its Derivatives

Bread and Bakery Products

The quintessential gluten carrier, bread is a staple in many cultures worldwide. From baguettes to sourdough, wheat-based breads are loved for their diverse textures and flavors. Most bakery items are among the most prevalent sources of gluten. Wheat flour serves as the foundation for these staples. Additionally, pizza dough, won-ton, croissants, pancakes, and waffles fall into this category.

Pasta

Traditional wheat-based pasta, such as spaghetti, penne, and fusilli are just a few examples of gluten-rich pasta varieties. *However, gluten-free alternatives made from rice, corn, or quinoa are widely available for those with dietary restrictions.*

Breakfast Cereal

Many breakfast cereals contain wheat, barley, or rye. It's essential to scrutinize labels, as even seemingly harmless cereals may include gluten-based ingredients. *Fortunately, gluten-free alternatives are widely available for those with dietary restrictions.*

Flour

Flour is a versatile ingredient, but common wheat flour is a no-go for those avoiding gluten. *Opt for gluten-free flours like rice, almond, oats, tapioca, millet, chickpea, or coconut flour as alternatives.*

Barley and Rye Products

Beer

Traditional beer is brewed using barley, making it a gluten-rich beverage. *Fortunately, gluten-free beers made from alternative grains like sorghum or rice are available for those who enjoy a cold brew.*

Whiskey

Certain distilled spirits, like whiskey, may be derived from grains containing gluten. However, the distillation process often removes gluten, and some people with gluten sensitivities find they can tolerate distilled spirits. As always, individual tolerance varies, so it's advisable to exercise caution.

Surprising Hidden Sources of Gluten

Sauces, Gravies and Condiments

Soy sauce and hoisin sauce contain gluten, as do some salad dressings. *For gluten-free alternatives, tamari sauce or gluten-free soy sauce can be used in its place.*

Thickening agents like flour are commonly used in sauces and gravies, making them potential sources of hidden gluten. It's crucial to read labels carefully or opt for gluten-free alternatives. Opt for gluten-free alternatives or make your own sauces at home to ensure they are safe. *If needed, use an alternative gluten-free flour or arrowroot for thickening gravies.*

Processed Foods

Prepackaged and processed foods often contain hidden gluten, including soups, sauces, and some frozen meals. Careful label reading is crucial when selecting these items.

Communal Fryers

Foods labeled as gluten-free may be contaminated if fried in the same oil as gluten-containing items. Be cautious when dining out and inquire about dedicated fryers. People have various sensitivities to the fryer contaminants. Some are not affected at all, others get the same symptoms as if they had eaten gluten directly.

Understanding the prevalence of gluten in common foods is essential for individuals managing gluten-related disorders. As awareness of gluten sensitivities grows, so does the availability of gluten-free alternatives, making it easier for individuals to navigate a diverse and flavorful world of food while respecting their dietary needs.

Chapter 4 - What is Gluten Cross-Contamination?

Gluten cross-contamination is a critical concern for individuals with gluten sensitivity, celiac disease, or wheat allergy. This chapter delves into the nuances of gluten cross-contamination, exploring what it is, how it occurs, and its potential impact on those who must strictly adhere to a gluten-free lifestyle.

Understanding Gluten: A Brief Recap

Gluten is a protein composite found in wheat and related grains such as barley and rye. For those with celiac disease or gluten sensitivity, **even minute traces of gluten can trigger adverse reactions**, damaging the small intestine and leading to various health issues.

Defining Gluten Cross-Contamination

Cross-contamination refers to the unintentional transfer of gluten from one surface or food item to another, leading to the contamination of an otherwise gluten-free product. This can happen at any stage of food production, processing, handling, preparation, or serving.

Something as simple as using a spoon or knife on first a gluten-containing product and then using that same utensil on the gluten-free item will cause cross-contamination and will likely make your friend sick.

A common example of this happening is at say a party. Someone takes a scoop of dip or butter and spreads it on a piece of gluten-containing bread or cracker, and puts the spoon or knife back down on the table. Then the friend with the gluten allergy picks up that spoon or knife and does the same but on their own gluten-free (GF) piece of bread or cracker. This friend has just ingested gluten and will likely feel the effects one way or another.

For individuals with celiac disease, even a tiny amount of gluten can trigger an immune response, leading to damage to the lining of the small intestine. Symptoms may include abdominal pain, bloating, diarrhea, fatigue, and malabsorption of nutrients. In the long term, untreated celiac disease can lead to severe complications. People with gluten sensitivity can experience a range of symptoms, including gastrointestinal, neurological, and skin issues.

Here are other ways cross-contamination happens:

Shared Equipment and Utensils:
In food processing facilities or kitchens, shared equipment or utensils that have been used to handle gluten-containing ingredients can pose a significant risk. Even thorough cleaning may not eliminate all traces of gluten. For example, a food processing factory runs wheat through a processor. Then uses

the same machine to process oats or nuts. Even if that machine has been cleaned before each type of food is sent through it, there will likely still be traces of gluten that can be transferred to the oats or nuts. If the packaging says "produced on shared equipment with wheat", do not use this product with your gluten-sensitive friend.

Shared Cooking Surfaces:

When a grill, oven, or stovetop is used for both gluten-free and gluten-containing items without proper cleaning, it can result in cross-contamination. Residual gluten from previous use can linger and transfer to subsequent dishes. For example, a wok that is typically used with regular soy sauce will contaminate subsequent food prepared in that same wok, even if it's been thoroughly cleaned and no regular soy sauce is used in that particular dish. *An alternative to soy sauce is tamari, which tastes the same as soy sauce but is gluten-free.*

Airborne Contamination:

Flour and other gluten-containing ingredients can become airborne during cooking or baking, settling on surfaces and contaminating nearby gluten-free items.

Bulk Bin Shopping:

Bulk bins at grocery stores where gluten-free products are displayed alongside gluten-containing ones may expose gluten-free items to contaminants. Customers using the same scoop for different bins can inadvertently introduce gluten. People with any kind of gluten sensitivity would do well to avoid bulk bin shopping. It is simply too difficult to monitor the safety.

Creating a Gluten-Friendly Environment

Dedicated Kitchen Tools: A typical household that includes people with and without a gluten allergy is best served by establishing dedicated kitchen tools that are only used for gluten-free ingredients. Many homes have two toasters, for example, and separate cutting boards.

Clean and Sanitize:

Thoroughly clean surfaces, utensils, and equipment before preparing gluten-free meals. Pay special attention to areas that may trap gluten particles.

Education and Communication:

Educate those in your household or kitchen staff about the importance of preventing cross-contamination. Clear communication is crucial to maintaining a safe gluten-free environment.

Choose Certified Gluten-Free Products:

Look for products with gluten-free certification, indicating that they meet strict standards for gluten content and cross-contamination prevention. We are fortunate that there now are so many quality alternatives to choose from.

Safe Environment Summary

Navigating a gluten-free lifestyle requires diligence and awareness, especially regarding gluten cross-contamination. By understanding the potential sources and implementing preventive measures, individuals can take control of their health and enjoy a safe, gluten-free diet. Awareness within the food industry, coupled with ongoing research, continues to enhance our understanding and management of gluten-related disorders.

Chapter 5 - Socializing

Attending a Party at a Gluten-Free Friend's House

Supporting a gluten-free friend at a party is considerate, and there are several things you can do to make sure they feel comfortable and appreciated.

Going to Your Gluten-Free Friend's Home

When going to the home of a person with a gluten disorder, please consider the following suggestions when contributing a dish to the festivities and while enjoying the food at the party.

Your Contribution To The Party

Please only bring completely gluten-free items. Whether you are making a dish or buying packaged items, such as chips, dips, or desserts, be 100% sure there are no gluten-containing ingredients.

You may be craving a delicious traditional baguette to serve with your dips, but the chance of cross-contamination is virtually guaranteed. Even those with the best intentions can easily get caught up in a conversation and unknowingly use that spoon to spread the dip on their gorgeous slice of baguette. Then if your friend inadvertently uses that spoon afterwards, they go into the next day with whatever symptoms they tend to manifest. Consider that it may be worth you forgoing a bit of traditional baguette or sourdough loaf for this one night to save your friend the risk of getting sick from cross-contamination. Have an extra slice the next day, basking in the knowledge that your friend is likely having a good day because you didn't bring that delicious loaf of sourdough (or traditional cookies, brownies, cake, pie, crackers, etc).

Or better yet, bring one of the following particularly delicious alternatives, and you will be the hero! For baguettes and pizzas, try the brand **Against The Grain,** found in the freezer section of your grocery store. Go to **Bread SRSLY** online or in Whole Foods for the best sourdough bread products. Companies like these will change the way you think of gluten-free bread. www. againstthegraingormet.com or www.breadsrsly.com

Your friend may feel obligated to serve gluten-containing items and may have a plan for avoiding cross-contamination. That is their decision to make. Please do not make that decision for them. Again, the odds of them ingesting gluten in these situations are high. They may make a dish that is just for them to avoid this problem. If there is a mixture of items presented, perhaps suggest your friend serve themselves a plate of appetizers before everyone else so that they have their food before the opportunity of cross-contamination.

Your gluten-free friend will likely have their own strategies on how to navigate all dining scenarios. But if they are newly diagnosed, it will take them some trial and error to develop these strategies. And even then, the landmines will still inevitably pop up, even for the highly experienced. So the easier you can make it on them, the better you will all feel.

Just like you wouldn't use bacon grease in a vegan dish, don't bring gluten-containing foods to a gluten-free household. Your effort to accommodate their needs will be greatly appreciated.

Naturally Gluten-Free Foods

There are so many naturally gluten-free foods to choose from. Here are some great options:

Fruits and Vegetables:
   Most fruits and vegetables are naturally gluten-free. Fresh, frozen, or canned without added sauces or seasonings are safe choices.

Meat and Poultry:
   Fresh or unprocessed meats and poultry are gluten-free. Be cautious with processed or pre-seasoned meats, as they may contain gluten-containing ingredients.

Fish and Seafood:
   Fresh fish and seafood are naturally gluten-free. However, be mindful of breaded or battered varieties, as the coating may contain gluten.

Eggs:

Eggs in their natural state are gluten-free. Check processed or prepackaged egg products for any added ingredients that might contain gluten.

Dairy Products:

Most dairy products, such as milk, cheese, yogurt, and butter, are naturally gluten-free. However, some flavored or processed dairy products may contain gluten, so it's essential to check labels.

Nuts and Seeds:

Nuts and seeds, in their natural form, are gluten-free. However, cross-contamination can occur, especially with processed or flavored varieties, so it's important to check labels.

Legumes:

Beans, lentils, and peas are gluten-free. Canned varieties may sometimes have additives or seasonings containing gluten, so it's advisable to read labels.

Grains:

While wheat, barley, and rye contain gluten, there are several naturally gluten-free grains, including:

- Rice
- Quinoa
- Buckwheat
- Corn
- Millet
- Sorghum
- Teff

- Amaranth

Potatoes:

Potatoes in their natural state are gluten-free. However, be cautious with processed potato products, as they may contain gluten additives, such as thickening agents.

Gluten-Free Flours:

There are various gluten-free flours available, such as almond flour, coconut flour, rice flour, millet, tapioca, and chickpea flour. These can be used as alternatives to wheat flour in cooking and baking.

Always check labels carefully, as some processed or packaged foods may contain hidden sources of gluten or be at risk of cross-contamination during manufacturing.

Gluten-Free Recipes:

It is really not complicated nor difficult to convert most recipes to a gluten-free version. There are hundreds of cookbooks and websites devoted to gluten-free cooking and baking. If you are up for trying it, start with an easy dish or two, such as a cake or pasta dish. The alternative flours are very delicious. You may be pleasantly surprised to learn that most people will not even notice the difference. As mentioned before, tamari makes an excellent substitute for regular soy sauce in many of your sauces, salad dressing, and gravies.

Hosting a Party at Your House

Your friend will not expect a perfectly gluten-free environment when going out, whether to a friend's house or a restaurant. As mentioned before, they will have their own strategies for socializing events. But there are some ways to help them safely navigate a party at your home.

Communication:

Talk to your friend in advance and ask about specific dietary restrictions and preferences. Some people with gluten sensitivity or celiac disease have different levels of sensitivity or specific trigger foods.

Menu Planning:

Be sure to include gluten-free options on the menu. This could include dishes that naturally don't contain gluten or gluten-free alternatives for common party foods.

Check Ingredients:

When preparing food or purchasing pre-made items, carefully read ingredient labels to ensure they don't contain gluten. Many processed foods may have hidden sources of gluten.

Accommodate Cross-Contamination Concerns when Prepping Food:

Be mindful of cross-contamination in the kitchen. If you're using shared utensils or surfaces, make sure they are thoroughly cleaned to avoid any trace of gluten.

Labeling:

If there's a buffet or snack table, label gluten-free options clearly. This helps your friend identify what is safe for them to eat without constantly having to ask.

Separate Utensils and Serving Areas:

Use separate serving utensils for gluten-free dishes to prevent cross-contamination. And clearly label the areas for Gluten-Free vs Non-Gluten-Free utensils. Make sure that gluten-free items are not placed next to gluten-containing foods.

Ask for Input:

If you're uncertain about certain foods or recipes, don't hesitate to ask your friend for advice or clarification. They'll appreciate your effort to make sure the food is safe for them.

Inform Others:

Let other guests know about your friend's dietary restrictions, so they are mindful when using the various utensils.

Create a Comfortable Environment:

Make sure your friend feels comfortable asking questions about the menu or ingredients. A supportive and understanding atmosphere is key.

Restaurants

There is little you can do to control the environment when dining out at a restaurant with your gluten-free friend, but there are still a few things that will make a big difference in their enjoyment of (and safety in) the social outing.

Choose Restaurants Wisely:
Select restaurants with gluten-free options or that have a good understanding of gluten allergies.

Ordering:
If ordering dishes to be shared by the table, be sure to order at least one gluten-free option. When it arrives, let that person take their portion first, so that there is less chance of cross-contamination.

Inform Others:
Inform the restaurant staff about the allergy and ask about their procedures for preventing cross-contamination.
Encourage your friend to ask about gluten-free options, cross-contamination prevention measures, and alternative preparations for dishes. Many restaurants are willing and prepared to accommodate special dietary requirements.
Let other guests know about your friend's dietary restrictions, if necessary, so they are mindful when sharing food or making recommendations.

Be Supportive:
Understand that living with a gluten allergy can be challenging, and your support is crucial. Be patient and empathetic,

especially if your friend needs to check labels or ask questions about food.

Chapter 6 - Why It Matters

To sum it all up, being diligent and considerate about a friend's gluten allergy matters. And it matters a lot. Here are several important reasons:

Health and Safety:

Individuals with gluten allergies, especially those with celiac disease, can experience severe health issues if they consume even small amounts of gluten. It can lead to damage in the small intestine, nutritional deficiencies, and other complications. Being diligent about their allergy helps prevent serious health consequences.

Quality of Life:

Continual exposure to gluten can negatively impact a person's quality of life. It may lead to chronic discomfort, digestive issues, fatigue, and other symptoms. By respecting their dietary needs, you contribute to their overall well-being and allow them to enjoy social gatherings without worry. It is a well-proven fact that a positive social community contributes to physical and mental wellness and longevity.

Trust and Friendship:

Being considerate about a friend's gluten allergy demonstrates empathy and understanding. It fosters trust and strengthens your friendship. It shows that you value their health and are willing to accommodate their needs, contributing to a positive and supportive social environment.

Social Inclusivity:

By being mindful of your friend's gluten allergy, you create an inclusive atmosphere in social gatherings. They can participate more fully without feeling isolated or having to constantly explain their dietary restrictions. It helps everyone feel comfortable and included.

Educational Opportunity:

Taking the time to understand and accommodate your friend's gluten allergy can be an educational opportunity for everyone involved. It raises awareness about food sensitivities and allergies, fostering a more informed and considerate community.

Setting a Positive Example:

Your diligence in accommodating a friend's gluten allergy can set a positive example for others. It encourages a culture of understanding and consideration for diverse dietary needs, making social interactions more enjoyable for everyone.

Avoiding Awkward Situations:

Accidental exposure to gluten can lead to uncomfortable situations, especially in social settings. Being diligent helps prevent awkward moments and ensures that your friend can enjoy the gathering without worrying about food safety.

Conclusion

In summary, being diligent about a friend's gluten allergy is a matter of respect, empathy, and care for their well-being. It contributes to a positive and inclusive social environment while safeguarding their health and allowing them to participate fully in social activities. And it's not as difficult as many think. It just takes a bit of education on the topic and a commitment to doing the right thing. I believe you will find that it is absolutely worth the effort - and delicious too!

Resources

The Celiac MD. (2023, September 30). *Amy Burkhart MD RD:Doctor/Dietitian/Gut Health/IBS//Gluten/SIBO/Celiac.* Amy Burkhart, MD, RD. https://theceliacmd.com/

What is Celiac Disease? | Celiac Disease Foundation. (n.d.). Celiac Disease Foundation. https://celiac.org/about-celiac-disease/what-is-celiac-disease/

Gluten Free Society. (2024, January 22). *Gluten-free diets, food & intolerance info for doctors & patients.* https://www.glutenfreesociety.org/

Against The Grain. (n.d.). Products. Against the Grain. https://againstthegraingourmet.com/pages/products

Bread SRSLY. (n.d.). *Bread SRSLY - Gluten-Free sourdough bread, also Top 9 Allergen-Free.* https://breadsrsly.com/

About the Author

Valerie Hepburn discovered she had Non-Celiac Gluten Sensitivity in 2008. Since then she has educated herself on the very best ways to protect her health and live an active and social lifestyle. She maintains a 100% gluten-free diet and enjoys delicious meals every day with the help of her loving and supportive husband. Valerie loves to host parties with her friends and family (many of whom have their own dietary needs and preferences) and has learned through trial and error the best practices for ensuring everyone has a wonderful time, whatever their dietary restrictions may be.